AFTER REHAB

A Simple Guide to Aid in Lasting Sobriety

by Kathy Dion

Cover Art by Catherine L. Savage,
Painting titled "Your Path"

PREFACE:

This book is for anyone looking for long-term sobriety, or for helping someone else with theirs. This is my personal opinion of actions that need to be taken to tackle this endeavor. After working in the field of addiction for 20 years, I have seen these actions become positive choices that have helped the addict move on to being a productive member of society by growing and building the sober life they've dreamed of. Most people think when one leaves rehab they are "cured." Leaving rehab, unfortunately, is only the beginning of a long road of change and, possibly, unimaginable struggles that for the average person, is the norm.

However, there is hope. It is easy to give up on someone, or even yourself, but leave the door open if someone is honestly seeking to better their lives. Only if it's a crack, leave it open. For that crack can shine a light to the addict brighter than you can imagine, especially if they are hopeless and ready to give up! Suddenly it may seem to them that the long road ahead is filled with promise! You have to care! You have to want it, and the addict has to want it for themselves. And in wanting it, you have to do what it will take, step by step, day by day, until the addictive behaviors that have been the routines of your life are replaced by positive actions that propel you forward into survival, and then growth, until you finally succeed in having the sober life you deserve for yourself, your family and for those around you! And to the addict, you deserve it!

QUOTE:

"Look for the helpers. You will always find people who are helping."

Mr. Rogers

DEDICATION:

Thanks to all the helpers out there!

TABLE OF CONTENTS

CHAPTER ONE:

THE PLAN

Usually when one is in rehab their counselor works with them on their basic plan; when they will leave, where they will live and what their options are for employment, all the while ensuring the environment is sober. This is usually a temporary plan to at least get the person on their feet while they work on their future plans and goals. This plan was most likely already completed prior to leaving rehab, but if it hasn't been done, here are some pointers.

Hopefully, you and your loved one has started working on a plan prior to leaving rehab. If not, they better get to it quickly or risk the sobriety they've achieved so far by however long they've been in rehab.

Some of the plan is obvious, some parts not so much, unless you have gone through this before. The plan should include, but is not limited to:

1. A safe and sober place to stay while you get on your feet.
2. Where will the addict work? What are their options? How will they support themselves? These are all things

that have to be confronted and dealt with. Otherwise, the addict is setting himself up for immediate failure.

If the addict doesn't have a friend or relative they can live with while figuring out the answers to the questions in number two (above), there are plenty of sober living homes they can stay at temporarily or long term. Be sure to check these out thoroughly. Where are they located? Is there a bar nearby? Is it in an area where there is drug use or are drugs available that the addict can easily access? You obviously don't want these things right in your backyard. What is the reputation of the sober living home? Are they successful? A good rule of thumb is how long have they been open? Are there any media reports on them? In California, these are not licensed by any government entity, so you have to be very careful about whom you are giving your money to and make very sure it is a safe environment. Ask a lot of questions before securing a bed at one of these.

The addict can also come up with a list of short-term and long-term goals. What did they want to do before they went down this road of addiction? Did they have any goals? Dreams? Or is the dissolution of the goals or dreams part of what led them to a state of addiction? It is a well-known fact that most teens get involved with drugs due to boredom. Even if the short-term goal is to get a job! That's pretty important, so write it down. Nothing is too insignificant at this point. This can also be started on a gradient; short-term goals could be as simple as getting up early every day and writing a "TO DO" list for the day, or can start with taking care of themselves (shower, eat breakfast and start looking for that job)!

There are other parameters that should be set up in the beginning, but I will go over these further in this guide.

In dealing with addicts in the last 20 years, the #1 thing they stated that aided in their sobriety was having a solid plan when they left rehab!

ASSIGNMENT 1A: If you (the addict), or the person helping someone who is the addict, do not have a plan as of yet, here are some helpful hints to get started:

1. List any and all family and friends that would be willing to help you.
2. If there is only one or two or none on the above list, search online in the city and state you are looking for sober living homes or transitional living homes. Check these out for Reviews, and map them so you know where they are located.
3. Start calling the above list and see what your options are in regards to both.
4. List the best possibilities based on location and financial reasons.
5. Reserve a bed if going to a sober living home.
6. Include in your plan to go directly there once discharged from Rehab.

ASSIGNMENT 1B.

1. Write out five short-term goals.
2. Write out five long-term goals.
3. This can always be updated and changed in the future. But write down what you feel right now that you would like to have, what your personal goals are, and any family and career goals you would like to achieve.

"Betty, a recovering alcoholic, stated that if she did not have a solid plan prior to leaving rehab, she would've started drinking right away. Writing the plan and sticking to it allowed her to set her own parameters and gave her many tips to maintain her sobriety. "

– eight years sober

CHAPTER TWO:

CHANGE OF ENVIRONMENT

I take the viewpoint that, if at all possible, one should not go back to the environment where they abused drugs and/or alcohol. I understand this is not always possible if the person is returning to a job or career, or a family. Often times the addict has drugs and/or alcohol hidden around the house or in their room. Sometimes they even forget where they hid these items and then run across them later. This is one of the many reasons why they shouldn't return to that environment. Also, there will be "triggers" in that environment that will remind them to use, or remind them of something else related to their drug or alcohol use. Such as; if they used in the basement and they go back down there for some reason, then before you know it, the urges kick in and if not handled quickly, can escalate into an actual reversion. Another example would be if they had frequently gone to a particular bar or liquor store in their old environment and when they go back home they have to drive by it frequently it could become too tempting.

An addict will often say they got rid of everything before they went to rehab, but as a rule, this is not true. If you think of the frame of mind they were in prior to entering rehab, it was not to get rid of drugs and/or alcohol. Rather, it was how to hide those things so they would be there when they returned. As much as they want to get clean, until they do, don't believe much of what they say, or at the minimum, take what they say with a grain of salt. If they are returning to their home or place of use do a thorough search of the area, and I mean thorough. You pretty much have to go through everything. It might be easier to throw everything away as far as hygiene products and start over. Every drawer and piece of clothing will have to be searched, including pockets and seams of clothing. Shoes, soles of shoes, and any place you could possibly hide something. You will be surprised at what you find and where you find it. I wouldn't take this search lightly, as this is something that comes up frequently (an addict finding drugs they had hidden earlier). This will be one of many tests. How they handle this depends on the kind of day they're having, but it is best if they don't have to deal with this first off, or ever if at all possible.

Living with a family member in another city or state while they are getting back on their feet would be the best option. I also feel this gives them the best chance of getting through the early stages of sobriety.

The majority of recovering addicts surveyed (sober 5 years or more) stated that moving from their area of abuse, allowed them to start their life over in a safe environment without triggers.

ASSIGNMENT 2:

1. List any and all people known to you that do not live in the area (city or state) where you abused drugs and or alcohol.
2. If there is no one, list three possible cities/states you could live in, or would like to start over in.
3. Once these areas are narrowed down, start searching them for sober living homes or transitional living homes.
4. Decide which is the best option and call to reserve a bed.
5. Include in your plan to go directly there once discharged.

CHAPTER THREE:

GET PRODUCTIVE

It is essential for everyone to be productive. But it is vital that you, the addict or recovering addict, get productive immediately. Lack of production causes low morale and boredom which leads to sitting around contemplating your existence. Then, memories of how you handled these feelings in the past kick in, and when you have too much time on your hands, you will begin thinking. What will you think about? Most people will think about what they're going to make for dinner, all the things they have to do that day or that week or they'll plan their future. An addict will start thinking about all the "fun" they used to have when they got high, or perhaps that their life is too hard and overwhelming and then they will seek to "escape" so they don't have to deal with their lives or work to overcome the obstacles that long-lasting sobriety represents.

If they are living with someone, I recommend that person sit down with them every night and come up with a daily "TO DO' list for the next day. Maybe you have chores they can do in your house or yard work outside. Perhaps they can clean your garage or help you with all the things you've wanted to get done. Obviously, you have to trust the person with your belongings, so keep this in mind when coming up with activities for them to do. Working like this will get them productive and help them contribute to the household they are currently living in. There are no free rides, and as soon as they think they can get away with one, they will start slipping back into old behaviors. We all know where that will lead.

The above is done until the person finds a job. They should seek employment right away. What job they can get or should get is of little consequence. The point is that they get a job, and start it! This is only a stepping stone and does not have to be their ultimate career choice. It is important that once they start this job, they keep it. They get up every day, they show up, and they perform whatever tasks they are given. It is vital that they get into this routine and start becoming responsible for their lives and supporting themselves.

But now that they are making money, the temptation to spend it on drugs and alcohol will be there. However, they have to start somewhere. Again, if they have someone helping them, this person should assist them in planning where their money should go and what they should spend it on. As soon as they start working, they should be made to pay their own way. Start paying rent, pay for their own food and their own necessities. They need to start doing this to become self-sufficient and learn that it costs money to survive in this world and Mommy and Daddy or other family and friends aren't always going to be there to support them or bail them out. It is wise that they learn this right away. (If they haven't learned it already; everyone's situation is different.)

"Mark, a recovering steroid and meth user stated that had he not gotten productive immediately upon leaving rehab, he would've relapsed."

– 6 years sober

ASSIGNMENT 3:

1. Update your resume, or create one. Preferably, this has been done before you are discharged, but if not, there are plenty of samples on the internet.
2. Start searching for jobs on Craigslist or other local listings where you will be living.
3. Ensure that when you send out your resume or calling about a job that you give the correct date you will be available. You do not have to disclose you were in rehab, you can simply say you are currently out of town but will available to interview on this date.
4. The idea here is to get a job, any job, so you get productive and start paying your own way. Be willing to take what is offered, as this will at least get your foot in the door and give you a start!

CHAPTER FOUR:

FIND YOUR FAITH

I am not going to preach or suggest any particular religion. That is up to the individual. But I have seen many addicts regain the faith of their youth and this has given them strength. They will need all the help they can get in the coming weeks, months and years. Finding that faith or a pastor to confide in has proven very beneficial. Often, I have seen a person's belief get stronger after completing a rehabilitation program than it had been in years.

If you are not a religious person, that is fine. I am not stating here that you must have faith in order to have lasting sobriety. If you find faith helps you find peace, and then participate. If it's not your thing, that is fine too.

It has also been beneficial for recovering addicts to attend AA meetings or NA meetings. This gives you a strong, sober group to be a part of. It is usually easy to find many different meetings which means you can try out a few and decide which ones work best for you. If you are not a fan of AA, that is up to you whether you chose to do this or not.

I should also mention that sometimes there are unsavory

individuals at these meetings that are often there just for court; because they have to be there. Steer clear of these individuals, as they are often not sincere in their quest for sobriety.

The point is to find sober friends and groups to be a part of. Recently, there are posts on the internet for sober groups and gatherings that are free to attend. This is also an excellent way to involve yourself with people that are on the same road as you so you can help each other on the path to continued sobriety while learning how to have fun again without the use of drugs or alcohol.

"Debbie, a recovering club drug and meth user stated that if she had not reconnected with her church and faith, she would not have been able to maintain her sobriety."

- 12 years sober

ASSIGNMENT 4:

1. If you will be attending church, you can simply go on-line and search for the type of faith you are looking for under the church search in your local area.
2. You can also search for AA meetings in your area.
3. There are also usually activities to do with a sober group. There will usually be a list when you search for "sober activities near me." If you can't find any in your local area, try searching in a nearby larger city. This will give you some ideas of the sober activities you can look for. You can always start your own local group too!

CHAPTER FIVE:

ELIMINATE/BLOCK ENABLERS

First of all, let's define what an "Enabler" is. The word enabler comes from the word enable, meaning:

"To make possible or easy." In dealing with addiction, enabling is defined as, "Accommodating the addicted individual in order to protect them from facing the full consequences of their drug use." (According to a study published in 2013 by Lander, Howsare, and Byrne).

In other words, are you or have you in the past;

1. Ever helped them to get drugs by giving them money or other assistance?
2. Allowed them to use drugs in your home or immediate environment?
3. Paid their rent, cell phone or other bills?
4. Covered for them? Made excuses for them when they didn't make it to work or a family function?
5. Lied for them in other ways?
6. Repeatedly gotten them out of a difficult situation?

7. Paid for their mistakes? In more ways than one?
8. Ignored the signs and pretended all is well?

If you have done this, then you are enabling the addict to continue to use drugs or alcohol and, in the end, not helping them. This is a difficult situation to be in, especially when you care about the individual. Usually this happens with a loved one. You want to help them, and often times when they are confronted by a loved one in regards to their drug or alcohol abuse, they will blow up and deny first and then make threats. They won't see you anymore, won't talk to you, sometimes they get violent (depending on the substance being used) and even blackmail you into feeling guilty if you don't continue to help them. However, they will keep up this behavior with or without your help as they are an addict. So, continuing to support them will make it easier for them to continue down this path. They have to hit their own rock bottom for it to sink in, for them to realize they do need help and that if they continue down this path, it will only lead to more pain, suffering, and possibly death. Sometimes, unfortunately, this means they have to get arrested or live on the street or overdose for it to sink in that they do need help. This does not mean giving up on the individual. It means letting them know you will not enable them anymore, and when they are ready for help, you will be there!

So, STOP enabling. Get them the help they truly need, not by paying for their cell phone or rent or money for food which is all usually used for drugs and/or alcohol anyway. If you feel you can't talk to them yourself, get them on the phone with one of the many helplines that are available. If that doesn't work, you can go the intervention route. These are often successful at getting the person in rehab. In the end, it is up to the individual. You can't do it for them; only they can take the steps necessary to change their own life. And when they are ready to save their life, you will be there to help!

Another point to be brought up is this: who are the addict's real friends, and who isn't? This is not always black and white. Obviously, you don't want the addict hanging out with people that use or abuse drugs. Or hang out in bars or other places that can trigger the urge or reminder to get high or drink. But sometimes, people that are uninformed or not used to dealing with addicts can create problems unwittingly. This happens all too frequently. Some examples of this might be inviting the addict to a party or event where drugs or heavy alcohol is being consumed. Obviously, weddings and other celebratory affairs will most likely involve alcohol. You have to decide if it is an environment the person can deal with, is ready to deal with, or if they should take a pass on this particular invite. The bottom line is that nobody should bring an addict or recovering addict, into an environment that might encourage them, however subtly, to use again.

A big mistake that addicts make is to think they can use another drug, or drink, because that was not their "drug of choice." I believe this is a falsehood. If someone is a heroin addict and they start drinking occasionally, this is a slippery slope. It is only a matter of time before they revert back to the high they like(d) or abused, and alcohol opens the door for that.

While we are on the subject of getting enablers out of your life, I want to bring up another area of "friends." The addict or the person helping an addict must cut ties with all the people the addict ever used drugs or alcohol or even smoked pot "occasionally" with. It's not that these people are bad (although some might be), but if you are trying your hardest to not drink or use drugs, it's not wise to put yourself in a position of being around those who do, no matter what. It is too tempting. And someone who is not an addict may not understand that the addict is someone that cannot just have "one drink" or smoke pot every once in a while, or use just "one more time." It doesn't work that way. The addict knows this deep down, even if they don't admit it out loud.

"Billy, a heroin and pain pill addict, stated that had he not gotten several supposedly "close" friends out of his life and gotten his family to understand enabling fully, he would not have stayed clean for the last ten plus years. "

ASSIGNMENT 5:

1. Make a list of "friends" in your life that fit this description that came to mind while reading this chapter.

2. If they are not immediate family and you can simply cut them out of your life, delete their phone number from your phone and email contact list, and delete them as friends on Facebook and all other social media.

3. Go through your social media accounts and delete any other enablers.

4. Do this with your phone and email accounts too.

5. If any of these "enablers" are close family and friends that you want in your life you will have to handle them to stop enabling. Have them read this chapter, thank them for the help they have tried to give you, but let them know you need to help yourself and ask only for their emotional support, love and friendship.

6. Do this with each one.

CHAPTER SIX:

GET HEALTHY

After years of abusing one's body with drugs and alcohol, it is time to get healthy. I have found this to be a massive benefit for the addict. (Actually, it's good for anyone, not just the addict.)

Since the focus for so many months or years has only been "to get high," the addict has been self-medicating and ignoring his or her body. To this degree, usually, when one gets clean and is withdrawing, they start to feel for the first time in a very long time. They can begin to see the toll on their body from the drug or alcohol abuse. This usually requires some doctor checkups and dental work once they are withdrawn from drugs or alcohol. When the body has been repaired of any illness, one needs to focus on rebuilding it. Get the addict on a good nutritional program that involves eating right, and start them doing some physical exercise. Even if it is just walking a few times a week.

Many addicts realize they have done a tremendous amount of damage to the body and it needs to be repaired. Getting healthy and eating right along with taking vitamins and exercising can be a very therapeutic process. It feels good to get out and use the body and get it healthy again. You've come this far, handled your addiction, and are clean for the first time in however long. It is vital that you give yourself every opportunity to keep that sobriety that you have worked so long for. Repairing the body and keeping it healthy is important. When the body feels good from taking care of it, you feel good inside! In this way, you have a better chance of battling whatever urges or triggers you to abuse it again.

As I said earlier, it doesn't take joining a gym, although that would be great. But getting out walking, playing a sport or group activity with others, all of this will help with this important factor of getting healthy.

> *"Phil, a recovering heroin addict stated that exercise and healthy living was the number one thing that helped him stay on the road to recovery."*
>
> – 8 years sober

ASSIGNMENT:

1. Make a list of physical activities that you enjoy.

2. If you have not exercised in a long time, start out on a gradient and work up to it. Even if it's a short walk a few times a week, this will get you outside and you can build from there.

3. Work these physical activities into your schedule at least 2-3 times a week.

4. If you need to change what you are doing or need a new activity, do so. There are many physical activities you can do; play basketball, volleyball, gym work out, swim etc.

5. Find others that enjoy the same physical exercise you do and start partnering with someone. This will help you both stay on track.

CHAPTER SEVEN:

HELP ANOTHER/ GIVE BACK

I have always said that the best way to help yourself is to help another. There are many reasons for this. As an addict, you have not just harmed yourself, you've also harmed those around you. It is very therapeutic to help another. This could be someone going through what you went through, or just helping your fellow man in some way. It can also stop that whole attitude of "feeling sorry for oneself." There is always someone else who has it worse than you did, or do. Not only that, a lot of people helped or tried to help you along your journey, so now you can pay their efforts forward and help others. I don't necessarily mean just help addicts, (though that is always a good thing). You can volunteer in your community in some way, help the homeless, volunteer at the local shelter or get involved in other non-profit activity.

You, the addict, have gone through struggles in your life and come out on the other side. Use those struggles to help others in need, in this way you are using those struggles in a positive way. Not only are you helping others, but you are also getting stronger as an individual. It is essential you pay it forward.

"Louise, a crack addict, stated that her best decision was to volunteer and help others in her quest for long term sobriety.

– 14 years sober

ASSIGNMENT:

1. Look up volunteer activities in your area. This can be a homeless shelter, food kitchen, humane society, your local church, school etc.
2. Make contact and find out when they need help and find one that works with your schedule.
3. There are many volunteer organizations that need assistance and you can help them and yourself by paying it forward!
4. Do this at least once a week, or when it fits into your work/family schedule. Everyone has at least a few hours a month to help another.

CHAPTER EIGHT:

MAKE AMENDS

Being an addict, you have stooped to new lows to feed your addiction. One has usually hurt the ones they love the most when they are traveling down this road. It is essential you make amends to not only those close to you, but also your immediate environment and humanity in general. This goes hand-in-hand with the above chapter of helping another. While you are helping another, you are making amends.

You can also focus on paying back the many debts you accumulated through your abuse. It is crucial that you focus on this as it is vital that you take responsibility for your actions. I'm not talking about doing your jail time and serving a sentence. I'm talking about paying back all those people that bailed you out, paid for your rehab, gave you a place to stay and didn't give up on you. It is essential that you pay those debts back, not just for yourself, but for the many people that helped you along the way. Your parents, siblings, husbands, wives, children, coworkers, and society at large. Admit it; you broke a few laws (at least) along the way of your abuse, it is time to make amends and own up to your mistakes. It also goes a long way to earning trust from those that don't entirely trust you anymore (and why should they?). Every little damage you make up goes a long way to making you a stronger person, stronger as an individual and stronger in your sobriety.

How far do you need to go with making amends? Well, how long have you been abusing drugs and/or alcohol? How much damage have you caused? The degree of damage you caused will determine how many amends you have to make. You decide. And be honest with yourself. Don't shortchange your sobriety.

Making amends goes a long way to helping you feel good about yourself again. You will reach a point where you feel you have made amends. This could take months, or years. But it can be done; it is up to you to keep up your hard work and repair the damage done.

> *"Bob – an alcoholic and pill abuser, stated that had he not made amends for his life of abuse, he would not have remained sober as the long-term effects of his transgressions made it impossible for him to feel good about himself again and thus forgive himself."*
>
> – 15 years sober

ASSIGNMENT:

1. Make a list of family and friends that helped you the most.

2. Beside each individual person's name write down what you can do to help them, you might want to ask them what they need help with as it may not be what you are thinking. The point is, you want to do the thing that actually helps them the most. You may not be able to pay back the money you owe them right away (if you owe them cash), but you can certainly help them clean their house, do their laundry, do yard work or whatever project they need help with. It is vital that you start doing this immediately. You will start to feel better, too!

CHAPTER NINE:

TRUST IS EARNED

It is essential for the addict and those around him to realize that just because the addict is clean and sober for the first time in a long time, they aren't out of the woods yet. Trust is a tricky thing. You want to trust the individual, but it has to be earned. Trust should not be given lightly. This is a vital step that, if ignored, can result in failure.

It is crucial that parameters are set up in the very beginning. Whether you are going back to live with family or a loved one or with a friend, these parameters need to be set up. To the reader who is helping another, what is meant by this is, don't give too much too soon. Set up rules that must be followed before the addict returns home. Guidelines for him or her to follow. Such as checking in regularly with a loved one and making strict curfews as to when the individual should be home as well as other rules for the household he is living in. You can pretty much set up anything you want or feel will aid in his or her sobriety. You are helping this individual, taking a chance, and trusting he will follow these rules and guidelines. He should willingly follow them for the sake of all. He or she can always make other arrangements if they feel they are too overbearing. The bottom line is they should be grateful you are still helping them.

One parameter that should be set up right away is random drug testing. This can be done at a local doctor's office, but is cheaper if you do the drug test at home. These can be purchased at your local pharmacy. You should do random testing, not the same day and time each week. As I said, you want to trust him or her, but until the trust is earned, unfortunately, you can't. You will need to go to the bathroom with them and watch as they collect the urine sample since it can't be contaminated or manipulated.

It is also vital that they get no more "free rides." They have gotten a lot of help and support along the way, and this is great. Help and support does not always mean paying their bills or phone plan or supporting them forever. A lot of folks want to help their loved one but don't know how. They think the only way is to help monetarily. This is not true; you can help by just being there and giving them love and support. It is essential that they start paying their own way, supporting themselves and learning or re-learning how to take care of themselves, their family and their future. It is time for them to step up to the plate and take charge of their life and start helping not only themselves but those around them.

> *"Tom, a pain pill abuser, stated that had his family not set up stiff parameters when he returned home he would've dropped back into old behaviors and started abusing pills again. "*
>
> – 5 years sober

31

ASSIGNMENT:

1. Random drug testing should be put in place. As mentioned earlier, these tests should be bought prior to the addict returning home. Have several on hand. You can do drug testing randomly (and you should) or you can do them when they come home past curfew or can't be contacted for a reasonable period of time.

2. Don't allow the addict to change the rules once home. If they become combative or do not want to follow the rules agreed to, you will have to toughen up and tell them they have to find another place to live. DO NOT BEND on this. If you feel there is non-optimum behavior going on, trust your instincts and drug test them. Sit them down and go over the guidelines again and tell them you will give them one more chance if you are willing to do so. You can also apply the 3-strike rule. He or she breaks the rules three times and they are no longer welcome in your home; they will have to make other arrangements immediately. Set a deadline and stick with this.

3. Once the addict has abided by the rules for several weeks or months, you can ease up on the rules. Do this one at a time and see how they do before you allow them too much freedom. This is for your benefit as well as the addict's.

4. Eventually they will earn the trust back, but this takes time, and it takes them actually showing you and themselves that they are sincere in maintaining their sobriety. This is done by following the rules, getting a

job and contributing to the household.

5. You also can and should set a time limit on how long you are willing to help them while they are getting on their feet. This should be shared in the beginning so that goals are set and met along the way.

CHAPTER TEN:

YOUR DAILY HAPPY

I feel an essential part of recovery, and for anyone else, is to discover what gives them pleasure and happiness and incorporate this into their life on a daily basis. It doesn't have to always take hours away from your busy day, but it is essential!

Wherever or in whatever you find joy, take a few moments out of your day and just enjoy it! Whether it be a hobby, a walk, exercise, gardening, reading or what have you. Even if you feel you are incompetent at something like painting, for example, who cares! If it gives you joy, do it! Take the time for yourself and feel that joy, whatever feeds your soul! This may sound silly or not important, but it can be the driving force that makes a dreary or busy day into one that fulfills you.

If you don't know what brings you joy, try different things until you find something you enjoy and then start incorporating it into your life. I can't say enough about this or stress it enough. Sometimes you can find someone to do these things with and sometimes this is your alone time to just be by yourself.

"Gus, an abuser of a multitude of drugs, stated that had he not actually found out what he enjoyed doing in life, which for him was returning to music, he wouldn't have found the strength to remain clean and sober."

– five years sober

ASSIGNMENT:

1. Make a list of things you enjoy doing: reading, writing, some type of exercise, a walk on the beach, whatever you enjoy!

2. Some of the things may take a lot of time and may not be able to be done on a daily basis and may be something you do monthly! However, there are other things you can incorporate into your daily life like taking a short walk, playing with your dog, gardening, whatever it may be. It is important you take a few minutes for "you" on a daily basis. It's important to bring joy into your life! It balances out everything else!

SUMMARY:

This is, by far, not all that goes into lasting sobriety. However, it is meant to be a simple guidebook to get you on the road to making the right choices for yourself, your family and for those around you. If you hit a road block or stumble a bit, (such as drink alcohol or use again) take a quick look at your life and see where you went into agreement with this behavior with yourself and or others. Remedy this immediately. Push through the molasses. Make the needed change and move forward. You can get back on track and take control of your life once again. Learn from the mistake and don't let it happen again. I wish you and your loved ones the life you want, filled with happiness, joy and love! So, take advantage of this time and live it fully sober!

www.ingramcontent.com/pod-product-compliance
Lightning Source LLC
Chambersburg PA
CBHW022135280326
41933CB00007B/701